Frequently Asked Questions

all about
SAM-e

DALLAS CLOUATRE, PhD

AVERY PUBLISHING GROUP

Garden City Park • New York

Series cover designer: Eric Macaluso
Cover image courtesy of Barry Axelrod Studios

Avery Publishing Group, Inc.
120 Old Broadway, Garden City Park, NY 11040
1-800-548-5757 or visit us at www.averypublishing.com

ISBN: 1-58333-021-6

Copyright © 1999 by Dallas Clouatre, PhD

Printed in the United States of America

10   9   8   7   6   5   4   3   2

Contents

Introduction

Although S-adenosyl-L-methionine (SAM-e) has only recently started making headlines in the United States, in Europe this versatile substance has long been considered a breakthrough treatment for depression and osteoarthritis. In addition, numerous studies conducted over the past twenty years have demonstrated SAM-e's ability to improve liver health, reduce the pain experienced with fibromyalgia and migraine headaches, and improve age-related brain disorders. In all of these studies, SAM-e (pronounced "Sammy") was shown to be remarkably safe. Of particular importance is the fact that SAM-e is not a drug. It's a naturally occurring compound produced by your body that is of direct importance to the proper functioning of numerous body processes. Years of research have gone into producing SAM-e in supplemental form, which is now available for use in the United States.

Lately, this substance has been drawing the attention of many prominent American scientists. At a recent conference held in New York, scientists noted that supplementing with SAM-e may help improve mood, joint mobility, and liver health. In light of the research studies covered at the conference, SAM-e was noted to be comparable in action to conventional medications currently in widespread use, such as common antidepressants and anti-inflammatories. Furthermore, one of the speakers at the conference pointed out that SAM-e doesn't merely cover up the symptoms of osteoarthritis; it may actually work to repair the damage causing the pain.

Your body produces SAM-e by combining the essential amino acid methionine and adenosine triphosphate (ATP)—the body's primary energy molecule. In this state, SAM-e, which is sometimes called "active methionine," is readily available for use in various body processes, including methylation. Methylation is one of the ways in which your body transforms compounds into other compounds that it needs to function. In this case, SAM-e acts as a methyl donor, contributing a methyl group (a unit of organic chemical compounds) to create new substances needed by your body. However, as you age and in certain disease states, your body may not produce the amount of SAM-e it needs to function optimally. That's where supplementing with SAM-e comes in.

In *All About SAM-e*, you'll learn about the discovery of this exciting supplement, how it works in your body, and why it's so important to good health. This book will answer your questions concerning the major benefits of SAM-e, and how to use it safely and effectively for beating depression, relieving pain, or boosting your overall health. Supporting scientific research will be explained in simple, understandable terms. You'll also find suggestions for SAM-e's proper usage as well as a guide to other nutrients to include in your daily regimen. By the time you finish reading this book, you'll know how to get the most out of supplementing with SAM-e.

1.

An Overview of SAM-e

SAM-e has many important effects on your body, including mood elevation, blood detoxification, and cartilage formation. Supplementing with this versatile substance has been shown to be beneficial in a variety of conditions, including osteoarthritis, depression, fibromyalgia, several liver disorders, migraine headaches, and learning and memory deficits associated with advancing age. But what exactly is SAM-e, and where has it been up until now? This chapter will explain what SAM-e is, how it was discovered, and why it is now being seen as an important element in sustaining the health of the body.

Q. What is SAM-e, and why is it so important?

A. S-adenosyl-L-methionine (SAM-e) is a compound produced by your body that is of direct importance to the proper functioning of at least forty major biochemical pathways (chemical processes in the body) and of indirect importance to many more. It is formed when the body combines the essential amino acid methionine, which can only be obtained from food sources or supplements, with adenosine triphosphate (ATP)—the body's primary energy molecule. In this state, SAM-e, which is sometimes called "active methionine," is readily available for use in various body processes. In one such process known as methylation, SAM-e acts as a methyl donor, contributing a methyl group (a unit of organic chemical compounds) to another compound to create a new compound that your body needs. Of the currently known methyl donors, SAM-e is probably the most active and efficient.

Q. How was SAM-e discovered?

A. SAM-e was discovered at the Laboratory of Cellular Pharmacology at the National Institutes of Health at Bethesda, Maryland, by G. L. Cantoni in 1952. Then in 1956, Cantoni and a coworker found that the synthesis of SAM-e involves methionine and ATP. The following year, J. Axelrod discovered two enzymes—the N and O methyltransferases—that play an important role in methylation. (See Chapter 2 for a discussion on methylation.) However, almost a decade passed before SAM-e was produced in a form that could be tested clinically. This molecule exists only temporarily in the body, so its production in supplemental form posed technical problems. Fortunately, these problems were overcome in 1973 by A. Fiecchi, when he discovered a process by which SAM-e could be stabilized. Then, in 1975, G. Stramentinoli published the first paper that explored the medical uses of SAM-e based upon actual trials. In 1976 and 1977 United States patents were granted that covered the production of SAM-e in the form of stabilized salts.

Q. Why haven't I heard of SAM-e before now?

A. There are many possible reasons why SAM-e has not become well known in this country. First of all, SAM-e is a natural compound that doesn't have the immediate effects of pharmaceutical drugs. Until recently, conventional medical focus in this country has been upon modifying the functions of the body rather than supporting or strengthening the various body processes so that the body can heal itself. In some areas the medical emphasis on intervention has proven to be highly successful. For instance, in a severe case of pneumonia, employing antibiotics may save a life, whereas giving natural supplements to strengthen the immune system will not work quickly enough. However, chronic conditions and age-related conditions sometimes respond better to supportive nutrients than to common drugs. For this reason, more and more Americans are turning to natural alternative treatments.

Most of the research on SAM-e has been conducted in Europe, which may be another reason why SAM-e has not become better known in this country. For decades, the European community has been much more open to nutritional and herbal forms of treatment. This openness has led to research into areas that have not received much attention in the United States. Quite a number of other compounds that are now beginning to be used in alternative healthcare were developed and prescribed extensively in Europe for years before becoming known in the United States.

Q. What's so special about SAM-e?

A. SAM-e is highly unusual in its ability to help

with so many different health problems. The benefits provided by SAM-e are equal to those of many beneficial supplements. For instance, SAM-e's been shown to be just as effective as glucosamine supplementation in cases of osteoarthritis, while at the same time providing the mood-enhancing effects typically associated with St. John's wort. SAM-e might be considered the equal of several powerful supplements rolled into one small package. Plus, SAM-e is remarkably safe and doesn't have any of the side effects normally associated with many modern medical treatments.

SAM-e can influence so many different conditions because its actions are directed towards a fundamental or underlying process known as methylation, which will be discussed in detail in Chapter 2.

Q. Can I get SAM-e from my diet?

A. The diet is not a good source for increasing SAM-e intake. There are a few reasons why very little SAM-e is actually found in the food you eat. First, in living organisms "active methionine" is produced only in small amounts for use in methylation and other reactions. Unlike enzymes, which are conserved when they are used as cofactors, SAM-e is used up through the loss of its methyl group. Second, SAM-e is a highly unstable molecule in the form in which it is found in living organisms. When meats are stored, processed, or cooked, SAM-e breaks down into other compounds. A great deal of scientific effort has gone into producing the stable form of SAM-e that is now available on the market.

Of course, dietary proteins contain methionine, and you may assume that merely supplementing with this amino acid or eating more protein would sufficiently increase SAM-e levels in your body. Unfortunately, this is not the case. Although exposure to a protein-deficient diet can reduce the body's ability to make SAM-e, eating large amounts of protein will not necessarily increase SAM-e synthesis, and can even result in a buildup of waste products, such as ammonia, which place an added burden on the kidneys and liver. Also, increased levels of methionine in the diet must be matched by increased intakes of the vitamins B_6, B_{12}, and folic acid to make its coversion to SAM-e possible.

Q. Why isn't SAM-e considered a vitamin?

A. Vitamins are very narrowly defined as a group of micronutrients present in small amounts in food that cannot be produced by the body, which are essential to life and health, and in insufficient amounts may lead to deficiency diseases. Therefore, vitamins are considered essential nutrients. Since our bodies produce small amounts of SAM-e, it does not fit this definition. In terms of function, SAM-e can be considered to have vitamin-like properties, but it is not considered an essential nutrient. There is increasing awareness, however, that many nutrients may be "conditionally" essential, meaning that under certain conditions, such as disease, stress, and aging, compounds normally produced by the body may be in short supply, making supplementing with the nutrient essential to good health.

Q. SAM-e sounds really great, but is it safe?

A. SAM-e is a remarkably safe supplement. The only side effects that have arisen as a result of taking SAM-e have been minor nausea and gastrointestinal disturbances. This occurred in only about 5 percent of the people taking this nutrient in high doses. In all of its trials, SAM-e has led to far fewer complaints than ibuprofen and other nonsteroidal anti-inflammatories (NSAIDs). In most trials, even those subjects who reported side effects did not find them severe enough to stop treatment.

2.

Methyl Donors

You've probably heard a lot about the importance of antioxidants like vitamins C and E for the prevention of diseases such as cancer and heart disease. However, the benefits of SAM-e and other methyl donors—substances essential to methylation—are probably not familiar to you. Methyl donors are very important for maintaining good health. In fact, these substances can help the body to defend against many conditions for which antioxidants are usually taken. For instance, in the case of heart disease, there is overwhelming evidence that improving the methylation process by increasing the availability of methyl donors will reduce the production of *homocysteine* (a toxic amino acid), and thereby reduce the risk of damage to important blood vessels. Methyl donors have also been shown to protect against cancer, reduce and repair damage to joints, protect against diseases of the brain and nervous system, improve liver health, and reduce the effects of the aging process. This chapter will give you a bird's-eye view of the nature of methylation, how methyl donors differ from antioxidants, and the many benefits of improved methylation.

Q. What is the methylation process?

A. Methylation refers to the attachment of one or more methyl groups (a single carbon unit with one carbon atom and three hydrogen atoms) to different substances to produce new compounds to be used by the body. Methyl donors, such as SAM-e (which provides the broadest range of benefits of all the methyl donors), have an available methyl group that is used in this process.

Methylation's impact upon the body starts at the most basic level—the expression, or activation, of deoxyribonucleic acid (DNA). Methyl groups attach to the DNA to provide protection against the activation of genes responsible for many diseases, such as cancer. Methylation is also important for the production of muscle-building proteins, for fat metabolism, for liver function, and for the production of neurotransmitters—the chemicals that supply signals to the nerves and the brain. For example, the transformation of L-dopa into the neurotransmitter dopamine, and the production of the hormone adrenaline are dependent upon the methylation process.

Our bodies are constantly transforming various compounds into other substances. Methylation is just one of the ways in which these transformations are brought about. In fact, methylation might better be thought of as the most significant of three related processes—*transmethylation, transsulfuration,* and *aminopropylation.*

Q. What is transmethylation?

A. Whereas methylation is referred to as the *attachment* of one or more methyl groups, transmethylation is often defined scientifically as the *donation* of methyl groups. For our purposes, the terms methylation and transmethylation are used interchangeably.

Transmethylation is involved in the creation of many substances. For example, L-carnitine—the substance that delivers long-chain fatty acids to the mitochondria (the cell's energy factory)—is created via transmethylation, or via methylation reactions. In addition, creatine phosphate, which provides the muscle cells with a quick burst of energy, is also manufactured via transmethylation.

Q. How does SAM-e influence the production of glutathione—the body's primary free-radical scavenger?

A. Once SAM-e has donated its methyl group in the process of methylation, it becomes a new substance called S-adenosyl-L-homocysteine, the starting point for the production of a number of important compounds in the process known as transsulfuration. Vitamin B_6 is a cofactor in this process. One of the endproducts of transsulfuration is L-cysteine, an important amino acid used by the body to construct a family of sulfur-containing compounds of vital importance. These compounds include the elements of the antioxidant enzyme pathway built around glutathione—a substance necessary for the scavenging of free radicals (damaging molecules) that are produced by glycolysis—the breakdown of carbohydrates for energy. The glutathione family of compounds and the amino acid taurine, which is another endproduct of transsulfuration, are important for liver detoxification.

Q. How does SAM-e help reduce pain and inflammation?

A. SAM-e is an important player in a third process, which is known as aminopropylation. This process produces spermidine and spermine, two substances that play important roles in cell and tissue growth. Another compound, methylthioadenosine (MTA) is a byproduct of the production of spermidine and spermine, and is part of the bodily machinery used in controlling pain and inflammation. Thus, SAM-e indirectly controls levels of pain and inflammation in the body.

Q. What other substances improve methylation?

A. Methylation is supported by folic acid, vitamin B_6, vitamin B_{12}, and the nutrient trimethylglycine (TMG). Of this group, TMG is the only true methyl donor. The vitamins act as coenzymes, or helpers, at critical times during the methylation process. Some of the functions of SAM-e require the presence of vitamin B_6, while others require the presence of folic acid and vitamin B_{12}. TMG is very useful in helping the body to produce SAM-e, but cannot perform this function in brain tissue. To a small extent, the consumption of the vitamin choline and choline-containing compounds, such as lecithin, is useful for increasing methylation because the body can convert a small amount of choline to TMG.

Q. What hinders methylation?

A. Just as there are nutrients that support the methylation process, there are "anti-nutrients" that can hinder it. Bad habits that place an added burden on the liver and almost always negatively affect methylation include smoking cigarettes, consuming excess alcohol, and eating a diet that is high in unhealthy fats and/or low in antioxidants. Birth control pills are another source of decreased methylation capacity.

Q. What's the connection between methyl donors and antioxidants?

A. Methyl donors and antioxidants have distinct, yet overlapping, functions in the body. Though they have different ways of going about it, both antioxidants and methyl donors protect cells from damage. Antioxidants work to control oxidation reactions. Oxidation is the reaction of a compound with oxygen, or whenever a molecule loses an electron during a chemical reaction. Antioxidants act by freely donating an electron to neutralize a molecule with an unpaired electron, also known as a free radical, before it can oxidize, or steal an electron from, the tissues of the body. In this way antioxidants, which are sometimes referred to as free-radical scavengers, help to control inflammation, blood vessel damage, fat oxidation, and allergic reactions.

Methyl donors can add to the body's antioxidant capacities, for instance, by increasing the production of glutathione—the body's primary antioxidant—as mentioned on page 20. Methylation also controls certain toxic compounds that are only slightly influenced by antioxidants, such as homocysteine.

Q. How does methylation influence homocysteine levels?

A. High blood levels of homocysteine, a toxic amino acid, have been linked to heart disease and to other life-threatening conditions. Elevated levels of this toxic amino acid may indicate sluggish, or inadequate, homocysteine metabolism, which may serve as a marker for decreased methylation capacities. When methylation is inadequate, there is risk of other health problems.

As discussed previously, the essential amino acid methionine and the addition of adenosine triphosphate (ATP) yield SAM-e. However, the body also converts some methionine to homocysteine, and then into homocysteine thiolactone, a highly toxic compound. Fortunately, with the assistance of folic acid, vitamin B_{12}, and trimethylglycine, the methylation of homocysteine can convert this compound back into methionine, which can then be converted into SAM-e.

The body uses SAM-e for most of its methylation needs. For this reason the methionine-homocysteine cycle must be kept working smoothly and efficiently, not only to reduce the levels of homocysteine, but also to keep the levels of SAM-e high. Homocysteine poses a threat only when the pathways to its conversion are sluggish.

Q. What are the effects of sluggish homocysteine metabolism?

A. According to the authors A. M. Miller and G. S. Kelly in a 1997 issue of the *Alternative Medicine Review,* sluggish homocysteine metabolism is associated with numerous illnesses. Many or even most of these diseases are not the result of the actions of homocysteine itself, but rather are the products of failures at the cellular level to produce adequate amounts of SAM-e and/or a failure in the transsulfuration pathway, which is discussed on page 20. Sluggish homocysteine clearance is associated with conditions such as alcoholism, cognitive decline, coronary artery disease, deep vein thrombosis, depression, diabetic retinopathy, multiple sclerosis, type II diabetes, impotence, osteoporosis, renal failure, and arthritis. More generally, various forms of birth defects, cancers, and liver disorders appear to be significantly statistically related to sluggish cellular homocysteine metabolism. With further research, even Alzheimer's disease might be added to this list.

Q. Are high homocysteine levels and reduced methylation related to aging?

A. Most of the conditions that are thought to be linked to sluggish homocysteine metabolism seem to be linked to the aging process. The methylation pathway declines with age, and this decline leads to a loss of the detoxification and repair operations that must be renewed moment by moment to maintain good health. Thus, supplementation with methyl donors such as SAM-e becomes one of the options that should be considered for maintaining sound health under conditions of stress and advancing years.

3.

Beating Depression and Improving Mental Function

If you or someone you know suffers from depression, you will be glad to know that SAM-e provides unquestionable benefits to people with this condition. There have been numerous clinical trials on SAM-e and depression, and in those trials that also tested common antidepressants, more subjects responded favorably to SAM-e than to the drugs. Also, SAM-e comes without the unwanted side effects of drug therapy. In addition to lifting depression, SAM-e also offers relief in cases of dementia, peripheral neuropathy, and migraine headaches, and perhaps improves other areas of brain and nervous system function, as well. SAM-e is unique in that it is the only methyl donor that has been shown to have the potential to increase transmethylation in the brain.

Q. What is depression and what are some of the symptoms?

A. Depression is a complex condition that affects not only mood, but also the physical body and its immune responses. Symptoms of depression include listlessness, feelings of despair, lack of sexual desire, difficulty concentrating, sleep disturbances, and eating disorders. Fatigue, digestive disturbances, and chronic infections are also common with depression.

Estimates vary, but approximately 15 million Americans suffer from clinical depression. Of those people between the ages of sixty and seventy who are hospitalized for other reasons, more than half suffer from this mood disorder.

Q. What causes depression?

A. Depression has both mental and physical causes. Events involving extreme stress, including divorce, the death of a loved one, accidents, or loss of employment, are common triggers of depression. Sometimes depression is the result of an illness, such as thyroid insufficiency. Unresolved internal difficulties are another source of depression.

Diets low in vitamins and minerals, and in some cases protein, often coincide with depression. Large amounts of sugars, refined carbohydrates, and junk foods are not sufficient to maintain good health. If the overall quality of health is poor, it is unlikely that mental functioning and emotional well-being will fare any better.

Two substances that are commonly found in the American diet that can undermine one's outlook on life are caffeine and alcohol. An intake of roughly 700 mg or more of caffeine per day (about five cups of coffee) is often associated with depression and mood swings. The consumption of excessive quantities of alcohol, especially before bedtime, can have similarly distorting effects upon mood. This is because alcohol consumption interferes with the body's natural production of melatonin, a hormone that controls sleep, and thereby disturbs the nature and restfulness of the night's sleep.

Q. How quickly can people with depression expect to feel the effects of SAM-e?

A. Depending upon the type of the depression, the dosage of SAM-e, and its delivery (orally or by injection), people with depression can expect to feel uplifting results within as little as one week's time. However, most individuals should give SAM-e supplementation a trial term of at least four weeks. See Chapter 8 for information on supplementing with SAM-e.

Q. What originally led scientists to suspect that SAM-e can help to improve mental functioning?

A. Interest in the role of methylation in mental functioning goes back several decades. In 1952, the same year SAM-e was discovered, a paper was published that hypothesized that some toxic substances associated with psychiatric disorders might be traced to a defect in the transmethylation of brain compounds. These compounds, such as epinephrine, norepinephrine, and dopamine usually act as neurotransmitters, and are collectively known as *catecholamines*. Researchers at that time suggested that such a defect can cause a buildup of psychotoxic metabolites—byproducts that cause mental derangement—in the nervous system, possibly leading to effects similar to those induced by mescaline—a drug that produces hallucinations. However, within less than a decade, researchers had refined their views and already suspected that it was not the production of psychotoxic metabolites, but a failure in the brain's transmethylation machinery itself that might be responsible for some psychiatric disorders. In 1978, when research was finally performed on schizophrenic patients to test this hypothesis, it was found the activity of two important enzymes responsible for transmethylation was greatly reduced.

Q. What is SAM-e's role in the brain?

A. There is no question that SAM-e is the primary methyl donor available in the brain, and its benefits in brain function are not in doubt. However, it is difficult to pinpoint any one brain mechanism dependent upon transmethylation that can be said to be improved by supplementation with SAM-e to the exclusion of the others. For instance, the neurotransmitters that might benefit from SAM-e include epinephrine, norepinephrine, serotonin, and dopamine. Many discussions about SAM-e focus on its effects upon one or more of these neurotransmitters, yet its impact upon brain function also depend upon many other indirect actions.

Transmethylation in the brain includes actions upon the special fats that are the primary components of all cell membranes. The best known of these in terms of its benefits to the central nervous system is probably phosphatidylserine (PS), a member of the class of compounds known as phospholipids. These compounds are often taken as supplements in the form of lecithin, but PS is not abundant in the normal diet, and is found only in trace amounts in the usual sources of lecithin. Supplementation with SAM-e improves the body's ability to manufacture phospholipids for use in the brain, thus providing important benefits by way of this indirect route.

Q. Is SAM-e useful in cases of drug rehabilitation?

A. Anxiety and depression are common factors in cases of drug withdrawal and rehabilitation. Mood-altering drugs typically work by unbalancing the production of brain neurotransmitters. Cocaine, for instance, temporarily increases the production of dopamine. Long-term abuse, however, exhausts the pathways to dopamine production and/or reduces the activity of dopamine receptors. Depression is one consequence. Because SAM-e acts to rebalance neurotransmitter production and receptor activity, it helps to normalize brain function. Abuse of opiates (drugs derived from opium) has unbalancing effects similar to those of cocaine abuse, although they don't involve quite the same pathways. In one test using 1,200 mg of SAM-e per day, former opiate abusers were significantly helped in their rehabilitation.

Q. Is there evidence that SAM-e can help with migraine headaches?

A. Perhaps one of the more surprising benefits of SAM-e is in cases of migraine headache. The pain-relieving effects of SAM-e appear quite slowly over a period of weeks or even months. Though the mechanism involved has not been explained, it's likely that improved membrane fluidity and catecholamine balance are important elements in this pain-relieving process. In many individuals, migraines are triggered by food allergies and/or by dietary amines (substances found in chocolate and cheese, for example), suggesting that liver function plays a role in migraine relief, as well.

Q. Can SAM-e help sufferers with dementia?

A. Dementia is a catch-all term for memory disorders, impaired reasoning ability, poor attention, and disorientation that can occur with the physiological deteriorations brought on by aging. The role of SAM-e in reducing dementia follows quite directly from the ability of this compound to improve the levels of brain neurotransmitters and their receptors. Recent research investigating the importance of SAM-e's role in dementia and its impact upon the various brain systems that might be involved found that SAM-e exerts beneficial and wide-ranging effects, though they have yet to be fully explained. Nevertheless, in other clinical trials as well, SAM-e has been shown to be of benefit against dementia.

Q. Does SAM-e have the potential to protect and heal nerves?

A. There is evidence that nerve health may depend upon the body's methylation capacities. For instance, in some inherited conditions, a reduced ability to produce SAM-e in the cerebrospinal fluid and in the nerves serving the extremities is linked to disorders in the arms and legs, disorders that in turn can manifest as problems in gait, locomotion, and muscle weakness. This is a form of peripheral neuropathy. Some published literature on this subject shows that doctors have been able to successfully treat this condition by giving their patients supplements to increase SAM-e levels. Other studies

have shown that SAM-e supplementation may help
the myelin sheath, or covering of the nerves, to
regenerate.

4.

Relieving the Pain
of Osteoarthritis

You may be surprised to learn that roughly 12 percent of Americans suffer from osteoarthritis, a form of arthritis most commonly associated with advancing age. In some cases, this condition can be physically debilitating. People with osteoarthritis and other joint complaints have become used to seeking relief by taking nonsteroidal anti-inflammatory drugs (NSAIDs), ranging from aspirin to stronger over-the-counter remedies. Unfortunately, NSAIDs do not show any ability to halt or reverse osteoarthritis, and may actually interfere with the natural healing process. Research suggests, however, that nutritional approaches may improve the underlying condition rather than simply mask the pain. In clinical trials, SAM-e has been shown to provide benefits comparable to glucosamine supplementation—one of the best alternative remedies for joint pain.

Q. What are the major forms of arthritis and how do they differ?

A. There are two major forms of arthritis, rheumatoid arthritis and osteoarthritis. Rheumatoid arthritis is characterized by inflammation not just of the joints, but of connective tissue throughout the body. As much as 3 percent of the population suffers from this form of arthritis, which typically surfaces in early adulthood. Most evidence indicates that rheumatoid arthritis is an autoimmune response that causes the body to attack its own tissues by mistake, leading to chronic and system-wide inflammation.

Osteoarthritis involves less tissue inflammation than rheumatoid arthritis, and is chiefly characterized by cartilage damage followed by calcification of the cartilage, the presence of bone spurs in the joint spaces, and similar changes. Primary osteoarthritis is usually considered a byproduct of aging with its associated decrease in the body's ability to renew normal collagen. Secondary osteoarthritis has a more direct cause, such as excessive use of a joint.

Q. What happens to the joints in osteoarthritis?

A. Osteoarthritis typically develops in three stages. In the first stage, the cartilage that covers the ends of the bones of a joint becomes chipped or cracked. Stress from excess body weight and/or overuse is usually involved to some extent, but the real issue is that of the body's reduced capacity to repair cartilage especially with advancing age. This results in rough cartilage that fails to properly facilitate the cushioning and sliding functions of the joint. Flakes of cartilage may be found in the synovial cavity, separating the joints, and synovial fluid may begin to leak into the non-calcified cartilage.

Stage two in the development of osteoarthritis is characterized by the development of deep fissures, or cracks, that extend through the non-calcified cartilage into the underlying bone, which evokes an unfortunate response from the body—blood vessels develop and grow out of the bone marrow into the gap. These vessels release clotting materials that plug the gap in the cartilage. However, the mere extension of the blood vessels into the non-calcified and calcified cartilage further weakens them because these vessels lack cartilage's rubbery smoothness and resilience.

Stage three in osteoarthritis is associated with most of the chronic pain and swelling so typical of this condition. The plug formed in the cartilage eventually wears down, reopening the original fissure. Synovial fluid leaks into the bone to form a cyst, and the bone itself forms swellings called *osteophytes*. Osteophytes can intrude into the joint and lead to a restricted range of motion and further damage the cartilage. Pain, stiffness, and difficulty flexing the afflicted joint are hallmarks of the third stage. At this point, the shape of the joint may change visibly. The synovial membrane can thicken and spread across the joint, further deforming it.

Q. What are the side effects of taking common pain relievers for arthritis?

A. Both osteoarthritis and rheumatoid arthritis undergo substantial numbers of remissions, or an abatement of symptoms, over time, especially if not treated with the standard over-the-counter and prescription anti-inflammatory and pain-relieving preparations. Research studies have shown that nonsteroidal anti-inflammatory drugs (NSAIDs), such as aspirin, interfere with tissue and joint repair. They usually do this by increasing the breakdown of protein and the loss of urea and sulfur, or by inhibiting the production of cartilage. NSAIDs also tend to encourage the formation of stomach ulcers and, with chronic administration, place an added burden on the liver and the kidneys. In fact, without the use of NSAIDs, remission from arthritis over a period of a decade can occur in 20 percent or more of arthritis sufferers.

Q. Does SAM-e work differently than common pain relievers and anti-inflammatories?

A. SAM-e exerts mild, yet beneficial pain-relieving effects. In animal trials, SAM-e has been proven to have definite anti-inflammatory benefits. In part, this may reflect the inhibition of one important pathway of inflammation products, the cyclooxygenase pathway, which uses arachidonic acid to produce highly reactive substances that can act as oxidants and free-radical generators. Moreover, SAM-e has been shown to increase cartilage formation, as determined by magnetic resonance imaging (MRI). At least some of the sulfur liberated from SAM-e during the process of transsulfuration is contributed to the sulfuration of glucosamine and to the chondroitin sulfates, which produce the building blocks needed for the synthesis of body tissues, such as cartilage, ligaments, and tendons.

Q. Is there clinical evidence that SAM-e can reduce the pain of osteoarthritis?

A. The benefits of SAM-e come through clearly in clinical trials. For example, in 1985, researchers at several Italian universities published data from a randomized double-blind multi-center clinical trial that examined the effects of SAM-e versus ibuprofen in 150 patients with hip and/or knee osteoarthritis. For thirty days, both compounds were administered by mouth at the rate of 400 mg three times per day. There were three times as many complaints in the ibuprofen group as in the SAM-e group. The researchers concluded that SAM-e was slightly superior to ibuprofen in the management of pain in these subjects.

In another trial, SAM-e demonstrated that it is superior to the NSAID known as naproxen. This double-blind placebo-controlled study of 734 subjects examined the benefits of these compounds for those suffering from hip and knee osteoarthritis. The oral dose of SAM-e was 1,200 mg per day and the dose of naproxen was 750 mg per day. Both compounds proved more effective than the placebo in reducing pain; however, SAM-e was better tolerated by the study subjects than was naproxen.

Q. Are there other treatments for osteoarthritis?

A. There are a number of herbs and nutrients that have been used to reduce the pain and the immobility induced by osteoarthritis. Glucosamine sulfate and chondroitin sulfate have received the most press, yet other substances may also be beneficial. These include the herbs and herbal extracts known as St. John's wort, Boswellia serrata, devil's claw, and curcumin, concentrated fish oils, the mineral boron, and the sulfur compound methyl-sulfonyl-methane (MSM), and another compound known as cerasomal-cis-9-cetylmyristoleate (CMO). There is no reason to try only one approach. SAM-e can be safely taken along with any one of these alternative supplements. Fish oils and MSM, for instance, typically provide a variety of health benefits, and therefore are usually positive additions to any diet.

In addition to taking SAM-e and trying other treatments, the chief recommendations are to lose excess weight and to exercise. Excess weight places stress on the joints and aggravates arthritic problems, and exercise helps to improve circulation to the tissues that supply nutrients to the joints. Moreover, mild exercise is usually beneficial for keeping the joints more flexible.

Q. What other supplements are good to take along with SAM-e?

A. SAM-e's benefits may be reduced if an individual is deficient in vitamin B_{12} and folate. Cartilage formation depends upon adequate dietary intakes of vitamin C and the mineral manganese. Boron also may be helpful. Therefore, for best results, these vitamins and minerals should also be included in the supplement regimen of people who have osteoarthritis.

Q. Can SAM-e provide some of the same benefits as glucosamine sulfate?

A. Although glucosamine, an amino sugar, is produced by the body from glucose, the pathway to its synthesis can be impaired and the demand for its synthesis can outrun the body's capacities. Therefore, the introduction of glucosamine sulfate, glucosamine hydrochloride, or N-acetyl glucosamine into the pathway aids in tissue repair by reducing the steps required for the synthesis of those tissues that are built from glucosamine. Most of the arthritic benefits of supplementation with glucosamines can be traced to the elevated rate of repair that these substances make possible. Research has found that SAM-e also encourages joint repair, but differently than glucosamine supplementation. Further research will be conducted in this area.

5.

Improving Liver Health

The health of your liver, one of the largest organs in your body, directly affects your overall well-being. SAM-e plays an important role in liver function. In fact, it is a key element in the liver's production of *lipotropic compounds*. These compounds are useful for processing fats and also for eliminating toxins, such as alcohol. Feelings of fatigue, poor digestion, allergies, and elevated responses to environmental toxins are often linked to inadequate liver function. Cholestasis—the failure of the liver to produce or release normal amounts of bile into the small intestine—is one of the conditions that benefits by improvements to liver health. In addition, SAM-e has proven its worth in cases of sluggish liver function and even in the very serious disorder known as cirrhosis of the liver.

Q. What exactly does the liver do?

A. The most obvious function of the liver is the secretion of bile. Bile goes first into the gallbladder and then into the small intestine, where it breaks down fat globules into smaller substances. However, the role of bile in the body is more complex than this, and is related to the liver's other functions as well. These can be divided between the storage and filtration of blood and the involvement in the majority of all of the body's metabolic functions. The range and significance of the liver's participation in metabolic functions can be represented by the fact that the hepatic portal vein (the vein that runs between the gastrointestinal tract and the liver) delivers blood directly to the liver before this nutrient-rich blood is distributed to the rest of the body.

Q. How can the health of the liver be improved?

A. Since the liver performs so many roles, it is critical that this organ be well cared for. This can be accomplished in three ways. First, the liver must be protected from the effects of the various toxins with which it routinely comes into contact. For example, bacteria and viruses produce toxins, and ammonia from protein metabolism is a toxin that is always present in the body. Various other compounds that are produced by the body, such as testosterone and estrogen, have many toxic after effects and must be inactivated by the liver. And then there are environmental toxins, some natural and some produced by modern technology. The former include the aflatoxins found in virtually all peanut products, whereas the latter include pesticide residues, dioxin from paper production and other sources, and the multitude of halogenated products (plastics) now found everywhere. Many of these residues act as synthetic estrogens and must be inactivated by the liver just as is true of natural steroids produced within the body.

A second approach to improving liver function is to encourage the secretion of bile by the liver and then the promotion of bile outflow from the gallbladder. The substances involved in this process are usually lumped together under the name of lipotropics. These can be divided between *choleretics,* or substances that encourage bile production, and *cholagogues,* substances that lead to the expulsion of bile from the gallbladder. Since toxins are often removed from the body via the bile, and the inability of the liver to detoxify properly can lead to the infiltration of fatty deposits into the liver, both of these approaches are needed to safeguard liver health.

The third approach to improving liver function involves adding substances to the diet that can aid the liver in its actions of transforming proteins, fats, and carbohydrates, in changing vitamins into their active forms, and in pursuing its other metabolic functions.

Q. How does SAM-e's capacity as a methyl donor improve liver health?

A. SAM-e promotes liver health by intervening in all three of the primary pathways known to be important in this regard. For example, SAM-e is used as a methyl donor by the liver to convert phosphatidylethanolamine into phosphatidylcholine (PC). PC is one of the best known and most useful of all lipotropics. Trials have shown that PC is very helpful to subjects with several types of liver inflammation, in cases of fatty degeneration, and even in cases of fibrotic damage, the thickening and scarring of connective tissues. Since many of the nutritive actions of the liver, that is those actions by which the liver changes or activates nutrients, require methylation, SAM-e has a clear role in promoting the transformation of substances.

Q. Does SAM-e supplementation influence the secretion and elimination of bile?

A. Several studies have examined the effectiveness of SAM-e in promoting bile flow and in relieving cholestasis—the failure to produce or release normal amounts of bile into the small intestine—and have found that SAM-e encourages the secretion and elimination of bile. This action may also explain SAM-e's usefulness in cases of Gilbert's syndrome. In this condition, bilirubin—a substance produced by the liver—is found in elevated amounts in the blood. A dosage of 400 mg of SAM-e taken three times per day has proven to be beneficial to those people who have been diagnosed with this syndrome.

Q. How does SAM-e improve liver detoxification?

A. SAM-e is a superb liver protector because its role as a methyl donor allows it to aid in the detoxification process. For example, it can help in the inactivation of estrogens—caused by premenstrual syndrome and/or the use of oral contraceptives—which are known to impair liver function. A number of trials have demonstrated that SAM-e is successful in protecting the liver and in maintaining liver function under conditions of excess estrogen. Likewise, animal trials have shown that SAM-e is important in protecting the liver against the fatty infiltration that can be induced through the excessive use of alcohol. Considering the fact that synthetic estrogens and alcohol are two of the most common toxins to which individuals in industrialized countries are exposed, supplementation with SAM-e might be viewed as a wise precautionary antidote. Some authorities suggest that SAM-e may be useful as a supplement during pregnancy to help the body adapt more successfully to hormone fluctuations and to the demands that these make upon the liver. Of course, if you are pregnant, do not take any supplements unless directed to do so by your physician.

Q. What is liver cirrhosis and how does SAM-e help?

A. During cirrhosis, the liver ceases to perform many of its detoxification and bile-related functions, and its regenerative mechanisms fail. As a result of this disease, the liver produces interlacing strands of fibrous tissues that constrict and bind the liver and reduce its functional capacity. Alcoholism, the obstruction of the bile duct, and a number of other conditions have been identified as causes, but perhaps half of all cases of cirrhosis have no identifiable cause.

Even in cases of cirrhosis, SAM-e has been shown to improve the levels of the antioxidant enzyme glutathione. Glutathione is one of two primary antioxidant and detoxifying enzymes produced by the body and is usually found in high levels in the liver. By increasing the body's levels of glutathione, SAM-e serves to increase the liver's ability to detoxify dangerous compounds.

Q. Can SAM-e improve the health of the digestive tract?

A. The evidence that SAM-e may benefit the digestive system is twofold. First, the health of the liver is a major factor in the health of the digestive tract. The flow of bile does much to control the nature of the bacterial balance found in the small and large intestines, and therefore removing cholestasis and other liver problems will have an impact upon the health of the digestive tract. A second line of evidence is the experience with other methyl donors in animal husbandry. For many years, it has been known that animals given supplemental trimethylglycine (TMG) have fewer digestive problems than unsupplemented animals. For various reasons, supplementation with a quality methyl donor improves digestion and stabilizes the bacterial balance in the intestines.

6.

Treating Fibromyalgia

The soft tissue disorder known as fibromyalgia afflicts roughly 10 million Americans, the majority of them women between the ages of twenty-five and fifty-five. As with many other conditions, fibromyalgia sometimes appears after an illness or trauma and other times may manifest gradually over the course of a few years. Once established, however, it tends to remain a chronic condition varying in degree. The usual sites of symptoms are the muscles and the insertion points of the tendons. Because the joints themselves are not affected, this is not considered an arthritic condition. In addition to the other symptoms of this disorder, depression is often common in people with fibromyalgia. This condition is typically treated with mild anti-inflammatories and pain relievers. However, studies show that SAM-e is helpful for improving not only the degree of pain experienced by people with fibromyalgia, but also their mood.

Q. What are the symptoms of fibromyalgia?

A. Symptoms of fibromyalgia include generalized muscle pain and aches, disturbed sleep, depression, fatigue, gastrointestinal disturbances, and tenderness at a number of anatomical points. These symptoms are often accompanied by anxiety and stiffness, especially upon awakening from sleep. It has been suggested that there is a close resemblance between fibromyalgia and chronic fatigue syndrome (CFS)—a condition associated with extreme fatigue—because there is an overlap in the symptoms associated with the two conditions. Some physicians distinguish between the two conditions primarily by the presence or absence of tenderness at eleven or more of the eighteen specific points associated with fibromyalgia. Both CFS and fibromyalgia tend to run in families, suggesting a possible genetic predisposition to these disorders.

The aches and pains that are characteristic of fibromyalgia are usually found in conjunction with constant muscular stress and tension in sufferers, and the inability to properly relax. Probable related symptoms include a heightened sensitivity to temperature changes, especially cold, and chronic muscular fatigue and stiffness.

Clinical examinations of patients with fibromyalgia have shown both abnormal circulation in the muscles and possible damage to the mitochondria—the cells' energy factories. This may mean that fibromyalgia is a state of chronic hypoxia, or oxygen deficiency, in the muscles, which is to say that poor oxygenation of the tissues may be responsible for the pain, fatigue, and stiffness. Because the symptoms are varied, fibromyalgia may be confused with at least fifty other conditions. Fibromyalgia tends to be self-perpetuating—a lack of oxygen causes muscle spasms, which prevent adequate blood flow, which result in hypoxia.

Because the muscle tissue is the usual active site of chronic pain in this condition, most research has focused upon muscle tissue. However, it is possible that the symptoms of fibromyalgia may be related to nerve tissue as well as to muscle tissue.

Q. What is SAM-e's role in the treatment of this condition?

A. SAM-e has proven to be useful for relieving several symptoms associated with fibromyalgia, including depression, swelling, and localized tenderness and irritation. Moreover, all of these symptoms suggest the possible need for supplementing the methylation process. And, if nerve health is, in fact, a contributing factor in this disorder, then SAM-e has even more to offer.

Q. Have SAM-e's effects on fibromyalgia been tested in clinical trials?

A. Researchers who have used SAM-e in clinical trials in the treatment of fibromyalgia have found it to be especially useful for reducing subjective feelings of pain and fatigue and for lifting depression. Clinical trials have tested SAM-e both in oral form and by injection. In a double-blind crossover study that tested SAM-e by injection in doses of 200 mg per day, SAM-e reduced the number of trigger points and areas of pain within twenty-one days in study subjects. The subjects also noticed an improvement in their mood.

Another trial compared treatment with SAM-e to treatment with transcutaneous electrical nerve stimulation (TENS)—a process that uses low-level electrical discharges to stimulate the nerves to lead to relaxation and reduced pain. In this study, SAM-e was given by injection in 200 mg doses per day and also orally to another group in 400 mg doses per day. The subjects receiving the TENS treatment showed very little improvement, while those subjects receiving SAM-e (in both forms) experienced a reduction in tender spots, lessened pain and fatigue, and improved mood.

Q. How much SAM-e should be used in cases of fibromyalgia and what should be expected?

A. The indication from one clinical trial that tested SAM-e in oral doses of 800 mg per day is that this level of supplementation is effective, but that benefits from this degree of supplementation will only become significant after at least five weeks of supplementation. As little as 400 mg per day taken orally has proven to be moderately effective, but the implication of these clinical trials is that either higher dosages or a longer period of supplementation should improve the results. See Chapter 8 for more information on supplementing with SAM-e.

7.

SAM-e's Other Benefits

So far, over 3,000 scientific research papers on SAM-e have been published. And SAM-e remains an important research topic that continues to attract scientific attention. More uses for this remarkable compound are still being investigated. SAM-e's effects on aging, immune function, and brain diseases, such as Alzheimer's disease, are currently being brought under consideration. Recent major scientific conferences held in both Europe and the United States have made SAM-e their primary topic of interest. Therefore, we can expect that SAM-e will continue to surprise us with new benefits in years to come.

Q. Does SAM-e have any effect on brain disorders such as Alzheimer's disease?

A. Methylation reactions in the brain decline with normal aging and, more dramatically, in diseases that affect brain function, such as Alzheimer's disease, suggesting a possible role for SAM-e.

Usually described as a progressive form of dementia and brain degeneration, Alzheimer's disease has no known cure. However, researchers have tested Alzheimer's patients to determine the levels of SAM-e and its byproducts in various areas of the brain and compared them with those of a control group. They found that SAM-e levels were severely decreased in subjects with Alzheimer's disease. This may be the result of an excessive demand for SAM-e due to an elevated rate of synthesis of certain brain compounds in Alzheimer's disease. That is, one of the pathways used to produce certain compounds may be overactive to the point of exhausting the brain's supply of the building blocks needed for proper brain functions. An important piece of evidence in favor of this interpretation is the fact that supplementation with SAM-e improves cognition and awareness in some people with Alzheimer's disease.

Q. Can SAM-e help ADD and ADHD?

A. Attention deficit disorder (ADD) and attention deficit hyperactivity disorder (ADHD) refer to a wide array of emotional, behavioral, and mental disorders for which there may be no single cause. Approximately 3 to 5 percent of school-aged children have been diagnosed as having one of these disorders. However, whether these conditions really have reached these epidemic proportions is open to debate. The more typical symptoms of these disorders include aggressiveness, the inability to concentrate or to sit still, moodiness, anxiety, distractibility, and even migraines. The drug Ritalin (methylphenidate), which is a powerful stimulant related to amphetamines, has the paradoxical effect of slowing down hyperactive children. Some authorities have written openly on what they consider to be the abuse of Ritalin. In 1993, the United Nations reported that the United States was already producing and consuming five times more Ritalin than the rest of the world combined.

The production of various neurotransmitters—including those which may be deficient in people with ADD/ADHD—have one or more steps in their synthesis that require the donation of a methyl group. Hence, it might be reasoned that methyl donors, such as SAM-e, would benefit those people suffering from these disorders. In fact, there have been trials that support this hypothesis. When scientists in Israel gave doses of SAM-e in oral form to subjects with ADHD, their symptoms improved dramatically. Another study at the University of California at Los Angeles similarly found that 75 percent of adult subjects who had been diagnosed with ADHD improved after taking SAM-e.

Q. Does SAM-e have any potential in helping to prevent cancer?

A. Methyl donors, as is true of antioxidants, have extremely wide-ranging roles in the body. Antioxidants are known to be important in preventing damage to cellular DNA, which can lead to the development of cancer. Methyl donors may turn out to be even more important in this regard. The protection of DNA, the primary substance of the genes, is an important aspect of methylation. *Demethylation*—the loss of a methyl group—is considered to be one of the sources of cellular decline that comes with age, and may be a source of the increased rate of cancer that comes with advancing years.

8.

Getting the Most Out of SAM-e

There is no doubt that SAM-e is a versatile supplement that provides an unusual range of powerful benefits. Very few supplements, natural or synthetic, can lay claim to so many significant clinical findings in such diverse areas. However, as with most supplements, it's possible to improve SAM-e's results by making use of synergists—nutrients that complement or add to SAM-e's effects. This chapter provides information on the nutrients that can be taken along with SAM-e to increase its benefits, and also provides you with information on SAM-e's appropriate dosage. In addition, a few relevant safety issues will be covered.

Q. How much SAM-e should I take?

A. If SAM-e is being taken for overall health rather than for a specific condition, 200 mg per day of SAM-e is a good maintenance dosage. The highest oral dose of SAM-e that has been used in the various clinical trials for depression is 1,600 mg in four divided doses of 400 mg each per day. The lowest effective oral dose used for depression is 400 mg in two divided doses of 200 mg each per day. There may be somewhat different responses to dosages depending on the condition being treated. Depression probably requires the highest dose.

For conditions such as osteoarthritis, fibromyalgia, liver disorders, and migraine headaches, an oral dose of 400 mg taken two to three times per day has proven to be effective. In some studies, this lower amount was useful for lifting depression as well. In cases of fibromyalgia and migraine headaches, a noticeable improvement may take several weeks of supplementation at a total daily dosage of 800 mg.

In one very large study, subjects with osteoarthritis achieved successful results by taking 400 mg of SAM-e three times per day for the first week, 400 mg two times per day for the second week, and 200 mg twice per day for the third week through the eighth week of the study.

Individuals should experiment to determine the lowest dose that is effective for them. Also, it is to be expected that there may be an initial loading phase—a period of time during which a higher dosage should be taken until relief from symptoms has been obtained. At that point, the dosage can be cut back, perhaps to as little as 200 mg per day.

Q. What nutrients can I take with SAM-e to improve its benefits?

A. Deficiencies in folic acid, <u>vitamin B_6</u>, and vita-<u>min B_{12}</u> may reduce the benefits achieved by supplementing with SAM-e. Therefore, it's always a good idea to supplement with these nutrients when you are taking SAM-e. For general health, SAM-e works well in conjunction with choline (250 to 1,000 mg), folic acid (400 to 800 mcg), vitamin B_6 (10 to 50 mg), and vitamin B_{12} (100 to 500 mcg). For cardiovascular health, SAM-e works well with trimethylglycine (TMG) (500 to 1,000 mg), vitamin B_6 (10 to 50 mg), vitamin B_{12} (100 to 500 mcg), and folic acid (400 to 800 mcg). For liver detoxification, SAM-e works well with L-methionine (250 to 1,000 mg), choline (250 to 1,000 mg), inositol (100 to 500 mg), TMG (500 to 1,000 mg), vitamin B_6 (10 to 50 mg), vitamin B_{12} (100 to 500 mcg), and folic acid (400 to 800 mcg).

Q. What are the side effects associated with SAM-e supplementation?

A. SAM-e is a remarkably safe supplement. The only side effects that are sometimes experienced with the oral form of SAM-e are nausea and gastrointestinal disturbances. Furthermore, these symptoms occur in only about 5 percent of those people taking SAM-e at the higher dosage levels of 1,200 mg to 1,600 mg per day. In all of its trials, SAM-e has always led to far fewer complaints than aspirin, ibuprofen, and other NSAIDs. Most study subjects, even those who reported side effects from SAM-e supplementation, did not find them to be severe enough to lead to the discontinuation of treatment. These side effects are clearly related to the dosage being ingested and, moreover, they tend to diminish with continued usage. Therefore, it is often suggested that people begin with a relatively low dosage of SAM-e, increasing it slowly until the desired dosage has been reached.

Q. How should the dosage be increased to avoid side effects?

A. It is suggested that SAM-e be started at a dosage

of 200 mg taken twice per day for the first two days. The dosage can then be increased to 400 mg taken twice per day on the third day, and to 400 mg taken three times per day after two weeks. If needed, after four weeks the dosage can be increased once more to 400 mg taken four times per day. Again, once relief has been obtained, it should be possible to cut back the dosage to 200 to 400 mg taken once or twice per day as a maintenance dose.

It is recommended that this product be taken on an empty stomach to improve absorption. Some experimental evidence suggests that the absorption rate of SAM-e may be increased as much as six-fold if the compound can be delivered into the small intestine without being acted upon first in the stomach. This would suggest that SAM-e should be taken via enteric-coated tablets or capsules because enteric coatings prevent tablets and capsules from dissolving before they reach the small intestine.

Q. Is there anyone who should not take SAM-e?

A. People who have manic depression (bipolar disorder) should consult a physician before using SAM-e. Manic depression differs from other forms of depression in that sufferers swing between emotional extremes. During the manic phase, there is excessive cheerfulness, even a sense of euphoria with delusions and a great deal of activity, but this "up" mood phase can quickly turn to irritability or aggression. The manic phase typically is followed by a period of deep depression. Lithium is the usual treatment for manic depression because it blunts both the "ups" and "downs" of mood swings. Manic depression needs to be diagnosed by a health-care professional and should not be self-treated. This condition is the only one currently known in which SAM-e may actually worsen symptoms. There is considerable dispute amongst researchers as to whether SAM-e taken orally, as opposed to administration by injection, will have a significant impact in manic depression. Nevertheless, caution is in order.

Q. Are there any known drug interactions?

A. SAM-e may speed the clearance of some drugs from the body because of its ability to improve liver function. No determination as to the significance of this has been made. Other than this fact, there are no known drug interactions.

Conclusion

By now, you are probably very impressed by SAM-e's diverse effects upon the body, which include lifting depression; relieving joint and muscle pain; improving liver health; and helping to prevent certain age-related declines, such as dementia. For years, SAM-e has been hailed as the European breakthrough against depression and arthritis, and has been the subject of continuing research in many other areas of health. Recently, this substance has sparked the interest of American scientists, and now SAM-e is available for use in the United States as a nutritional supplement. SAM-e can be taken for a variety of conditions without the side effects commonly associated with conventional medicines.

In short, SAM-e is a powerful nutrient that provides many benefits—with more on the way as research progresses. This incredible supplement can virtually replace a crowded shelf of individual remedies!

Glossary

Adenosine triphosphate (ATP). The body's primary energy molecule.

Aminopropylation. The process that utilizes SAM-e to produce spermidine and spermine, substances that are important for cell growth and differentiation, nerve regeneration, and more.

Antidepressant. Medication used to decrease the symptoms associated with depression.

Anti-inflammatory. A substance that reduces inflammation and the associated pain and swelling.

Antioxidant. A substance that prevents or controls oxidation by free radicals. Vitamins C and E are examples of antioxidants.

Atherosclerosis. A disease of the arteries in which plaques develop as oxidized fats penetrate the vessel walls and lead to progressive damage. When extensive, these plaques can narrow or even completely obstruct the arteries and cut off the flow of blood.

Atom. The smallest unit of an element, such as hydrogen or iron. Atoms become linked to form molecules.

ATP. *See* Adenosine triphosphate.

Biochemical pathway. A defined set of reactions by which a compound gives rise to other compounds in a living organism. For instance, transsulfuration is a biochemical pathway.

Cofactors. Substances that are necessary for the actions of other body compounds.

Cystathione β-synthase. The enzyme that converts the toxic compound homocysteine into the nontoxic amino acid cystathionine; SAM-e and vitamin B_6 are necessary for this conversion

Demethylation. The removal of a methyl group from DNA or other molecules

Deoxyribonucleic acid (DNA). The molecule that forms the basis of genetics and provides cells with instructions on how to behave.

DNA. *See* Deoxyribonucleic acid.

Enzyme. A protein molecule that increases the rate of chemical reactions.

Free Radical. An atom or molecule with an unpaired electron that can set off a series of oxidative reactions. Free radicals damage both proteins and fats in the body, including the membranes of cells and the DNA and the mitochondria within the cells.

Homocysteine. A toxic amino acid that is manufactured as a result of methionine metabolism.

Homocysteine thiolactone. A more damaging form of homocysteine, which is suspected of contributing to the development of heart disease.

Lipids. Fats and oils; lipids are found in all cell membranes and are used for both energy and hormone production.

Metabolic pathway. The steps or ordered pathway through which a particular biochemical process is accomplished. For instance, there is a metabolic pathway for the production of energy from carbohydrates.

Metabolism. Refers to the totality of biochemical processes of the body, or to the pathway and fate of a particular aspect of activity in the body, such as the metabolism of fats.

Methionine. An essential and nontoxic amino acid that is the building block for both SAM-e and homocysteine.

Methyl group. A unit of organic chemical compounds, consisting of one carbon and three hydrogen atoms. When attached to a section of DNA, it protects against damage to the genetic code; when attached to homocysteine, it converts the toxic amino acid to methionine.

Methylation. The process of attaching methyl groups to DNA, homocysteine, and other compounds in the body. *See also* Transmethylation.

Mitochondria. Small organelles found within cells, which produce most of the energy that is generated from food.

Molecule. The smallest unit of a substance that retains the properties of that substance; composed of one or more atoms.

Neurotransmitters. Chemical substances released from nerve cells to signal other nerve cells by activating receptor sites. Examples include dopamine, norepinephrine, and serotonin.

Oxidation. The process by which an electron is lost from an atom. An example of oxidation is the rusting of iron.

Transmethylation. The process by which methyl groups are transferred between methyl donors and methyl receptors. *See also* Methylation.

Transsulfuration. The pathway by which sulfur is removed from homocysteine to produce the amino acids cystathionine, cysteine, and taurine.

References

Adachi Y, et al., "The effects of S-adenosyl-methionine on Intrahepatic Cholestasis," *Japanese Archives Internal Medicine* 33 (1986):185–192.

Angelico M, et al., "Oral S-adenosyl-L-methionine (SAM-e) Administration Enhances Bile Salt Conjugation With Taurine in Patients with Liver Cirrhosis," *Scandinavian Journal of Clinical & Laboraory Investigations* 54 (1994):459–464.

Baldessarini RJ, "Neuropharmacology of S-adenosyl-L-methionine," *American Journal of Medicine* 83 (Suppl. 5A) (1987):95–103.

Bell KM, et al., "S-adenosylmethionine Blood Levels in Major Depression: Changes with Drug Treatment," *Acta Neurologica Scandinavica* 154 (Suppl.) (1994): 15–18.

Berger R and Nowak H, "A New Medical Approach to the Treatment of Osteoarthritis: Report of an open phase IV study with ademetionine (Gumbaral)," *American Journal of Medicine* 83 (Suppl. 5A) (1987): 84–88.

Bombardieri G, et al., "Intestinal Absorption of S-adenosyl-L-methionine in Humans," *Scandinavian Journal of Clinical & International Journal of Clinical Pharmacology, Therapy & Toxicology* 21 (1983): 186–188.

Bombardieri G, Milani A, Bernardi L, and Rossi L, "Effects of S-adenosyl-L-methionine (SAM-e) in the Treatment of Gilbert's Syndrome," *Current Therapeutic Research* 37 (1985):580–585.

Bottiglieri T, Laundry M, Martin R, et al., "S-adenosylmethionine Influences Monoamine Metabolism," *Lancet* ii (1984):224.

Brandt KD, "Effects of Nonsteroidal Anti-inflammatory Drugs on Chondrocyte Metabolism in vitro and in vivo," *American Journal of Medicine* 83 (Suppl. 5A) (1987):29–34.

Brooks PM, Potter SR, and Buchanan W, "NSAID and Osteoarthritis: Help or Hindrance," *Journal of Rheumatology* 9 (1982):3–5.

Carney MWP, Toone BK, and Reynolds EH, "S-adenosylmethionine and Affective Disorder," *Amer-*

ican Journal of Medicine 83 (Suppl. 5A) (1987): 104–106.

Caruso I and Pietrogrande V, "Italian Double-blind Multicenter Study Comparing S-adenosylmethionine, Naproxen, and Placebo in the Treatment of Degenerative Joint Disease," *American Journal of Medicine* 83 (Suppl. 5A) (1987):66–71.

Cerutti R, et al., "Psychological Distress During Peurperium: A Novel Therapeutic Approach Using S-adenosylmethionine," *Current Therapeutic Research* 53 (1993):707–717.

De Vanna M and Rigamonti R, "Oral S-adenosyl-L-methionine in Depression," *Current Therapeutic Research* 52 (1992):478–485.

Di Benedetto P, Lona LG, and Zidarich V, "Clinical Evaluation of S-adenosyl-L-methionine Versus Transcutaneous Nerve Stimulation in Primary Fibromyalgia," *Current Therapeutic Research* 53 (1993): 222–229.

Domljan Z, et al., "A Double-blind Trial of Ademetionine vs. Naproxen in Activated Gonarthrosis," *International Journal of Clinical Pharmacology, Therapy & Toxicology* 27 (1989):329–333.

Frankel P, Madsen F, *Stop Homocysteine Through the Methylation Process.* Thousand Oaks, CA: The Research Corner, 1998.

Frezza M, et al., "Oral S-adenosylmethionine in the Symptomatic Treatment of Intrahepatic Cholestasis: A Double-blind, Placebo-Controlled Study," *Gastroenterology* 99 (1990):211–215.

Frezza M, et al., "S-adenosylmethionine Counteracts Oral Contraceptive Hepatotoxicity in Women," *American Journal of Medicine Science* 293 (1987):234–238.

Frezza M, Pozzato C, Chiesa L, et al., "Reversal of Intrahepatic Cholestasis of Pregnancy in Women After High Dose S-adenosyl-L-methionine (SAM-e) Administration," *Hepatology* 4 (1984):274–278.

Friedel HA, Goa KL, and Benfield P, "S-adenosylmethionine," *Drugs* 38 (1989):3,889–3,917.

Gatto C, et al., "Analgesizing Effect of a Methyl Donor (9-adenosylmethionine) in Migraine: An Open Clinical Trial," *International Journal of Clinical Pharmacology Research* 6 (1986):15–17.

Glorioso S, et al., "Double-blind Multicentre Study of the Activity of S-adenosylmethionine in Hip and Knee Osteoarthritis," *International Journal of Clinical Pharmacology Research* 5 (1985):39–49.

Harmand MF, et al., "Effects of S-adenosylmethionine On Human Articular Chondrocyte Differentiation: An in vitro study," *American Journal of Medicine* 83 (Suppl. 5A) (1987):48–54.

Jacobsen S, et al., "Oral S-adenosylmethionine in Primary Fibromyalgia: Double-blind Clinical Evaluation," *Scandinavian Journal of Rheumatology* 20 (1991):294-302.

Janicak PC, et al., "Parenteral S-adenosylmethionine in Depression: A Literature Review and Preliminary Report," *Psychopharmacology Bulletin* 25 (1989): 238–241.

Kakimoto H, et al., "Changes in Lipid Composition of Erythrocyte Membranes with Administration of S-adenosyl-L-methionine in Chronic Liver Disease," *Gastroenterolia Japonica* 27 (1992):508–513.

Kagan BL, et al., "Oral S-adenosylmethionine in Depression: A Randomized, Double-blind Placebo-controlled Trial," *American Journal of Psychiatry* 147 (1990):591–595.

Konig H, et al., "Magnetic Resonance Tomography of Finger Polyarthritis: Morphology and Cartilage Signals After Ademetionine Therapy," *Aktuelle Radiol* 5 (1995):36–40.

Konig B, "A Long-Term (two years) Clinical Trial With S-adenosylmethionine for the Treatment of Osteoarthritis," *American Journal of Medicine* 83 (Suppl. 5A) (1987):89–94.

Loguercio C, et al., "Effect of S-adenosyl-L-methionine Administration on Red Blood Cell Cysteine and Glutathione Levels in Alcoholic Patients With and Without Liver Disease," *Alcohol Alcoholism* 29 (1994):597–604.

LoRusso A, et al., "Efficacy of S-adenosyl-L-methionine in Relieving Psychological Distress Associated With Detoxification in Opiate Abusers," *Current Therapeutic Research* 55 (1994):905–913.

Maccagno A, "Double-blind Controlled Clinical Trial of Oral S-adenosylmethionine Versus Piroxicam in Knee Osteoarthritis," *American Journal of Medicine* 83 (Suppl. 5A) (1987):72–77.

Marcolongo R, et al., "Double-blind Multicentre Study of the Activity of S-adenosyl-methionine in Hip and Knee osteoarthritis," *Current Therapeutic Research* 37 (1985):82–94.

Mazzanti R, et al., "On the Antisteatosic Effects of S-adenosyl-L-methionine in Various Chronic Liver Diseases: A Multicenter Study," *Current Therapeutic Research* 25 (1979):25–32.

Morrison LD, Smith DD, Kish SJ, "Brain S-adenosylmethionine Levels are Severely Decreased in Alzheimer's Disease," *Journal of Neurochemistry* 67 (1996):1,328–1,331.

Muller-Fassbender H, "Double-blind Clinical Trial of S-adenosylmethionine Versus ibuprofen in the Treatment of Osteoarthritis," *American Journal of Medicine* 83 (Suppl. 5A) (1987):81–83.

Newman NM and Ling RSM, "Acetabular Bone Destruction Related to Non-steroidal Anti-inflammatory Drugs," *Lancet* ii (1985):11–13.

Padova C, Tritapepe R, Padova F, et al., "S-adenosyl-L-methionine Antagonizes Oral Contraceptive-induced Bile Cholesterol Supersaturation in Healthy Women: Preliminary Report of a Controlled Randomized Trial," *American Journal of Gastroenterology* 79 (1984):941–944.

Pascale RM, et al., "Chemoprevention of Rat Liver Carcinogenesis by S-adenosyl-L-methionine: A Long-term Study," *Cancer Research* 52 (1992): 4,979–4,986.

Reicks M and Hathcock JN, "Effects of Methionine and Other Sulfur Compounds on Drug Conjugations," *Pharmaceutical Therapy* 37 (1988):67–79.

Reynolds E, Carney M, and Toone B, "Methylation and Mood," *Lancet* ii, (1983):196–199.

Rosenbaum JF, et al., "An Open-Label Pilot Study of Oral S-adenosylmethionine in Major Depression," *Psychopharmacology Bulletin* 24 (1988):189–194.

Salinaggi P, et al., "Double-blind, Placebo-controlled Study of S-adenosyl-L-methionine in Depressed Postmenopausal Women," *Psychotherapy Psychosomatics* 59 (1993):34–40.

Shield MJ, "Anti-inflammatory Drugs and Their Effects on Cartilage Synthesis and Renal Function," *European Journal of Rheumatology & Inflammation* 13 (1993):7–16.

Solomon L, "Drug Induced Arthropathy and Necrosis of the Femoral Head," *Journal of Bone & Joint Surgery* 55B (1973):246–251.

Stramentinoli G, "Pharmacological Aspects of S-adenosylmethionine: Pharmacokinetics and Pharmacodynamics," *American Journal of Medicine* 83 (Suppl. 5A) (1987):35–42.

Tavoni A, et al., "Evaluation of S-adenosylmethionine in Primary Fibromyalgia: A Double-blind Crossover Study," *American Journal of Medicine* 83 (Suppl. 5A) (1987):107–110.

Vahora SA and Malek-Ahmadi P, "S-adenosylmethionine in Depression," *Neuroscience Biobehavioral Review,* 12 (1988):139–141.

Vetter G, "Double-blind Comparative Clinical Trial With S-adenosylmethionine and Indomethacin in the Treatment of Osteoarthritis," *American Journal of Medicine* 83 (Suppl. 5A) (1987):78–80.

Workshop on Methionine Metabolism IV: Molecular Mechanisms and Clinical Implications (Consejo Superior Investigaciones Cientificas, 1998).

Suggested Readings

Balch JF, Balch PA. *Prescription for Nutritional Healing*, Second Edition. Garden City Park, NY: Avery Publishing Group, 1997.

Challem J. *All About Vitamins*. Garden City Park, NY: Avery Publishing Group, 1998.

Challem J, Dolby V. *Homocysteine: The Secret Killer*. New Canaan, CT: Keats, 1997.

Frankel P, Madsen F. *Stop Homocysteine Through the Methylation Process*. Thousand Oaks, CA: The Research Corner, 1998.

Grazi S, Costa M. *SAM-e (S-adenosylmethionine): The European Arthritis and Depression Breakthrough*. Rocklin, CA: Prima Health, 1999.

Lombard J, Germano C. *The Brain Wellness Plan*. New York, NY: Kensington Books, 1997.

McCully KS. *The Homocysteine Revolution*. New Canaan, CT: Keats, 1997.

Index